PERICONCEPTIONAL IRON SUPPLEMENTATION AND IRON AND FOLATE STATUS AMONG PREGNANT AND NON-PREGNANT WOMEN.

by

Humeera Rafeeq

TABLE OF CONTENTS

1.0		**INTRODUCTION**	1
2.0		**LITERATURE REVIEW**	3
	2.1	**Anemia: epidemiology, control and prevention**	3
	2.2	**Prevention and control of anemia in developing countries**	5
	2.3	**Risk factors associated adolescent childbearing**	6
	2.3.1	Maternal outcomes	7
	2.3.2	Infant outcomes	8
	2.4	**Iron**	9
	2.4.1	Iron metabolism	10
	2.4.2	Iron requirements among women of reproductive age	13
	2.4.3	Dietary sources of iron	15
	2.4.4	Assessment of iron status	16
	2.4.4.1	Hemoglobin	17
	2.4.4.2	Ferritin	19
	2.4.4.3	Transferrin Receptor	20
	2.5	**Folate**	21
	2.5.1	Folate metabolism	22
	2.5.2	Folate requirements among women of reproductive age	24
	2.5.3	Dietary sources of folate	25
	2.5.4	Assessment of folate status	25
	2.5.4.1	Erythrocyte folate	26
	2.5.4.2	Serum folate	26
	2.6	**Iron supplementation during pregnancy**	27
	2.7	**Folic acid supplementation during pregnancy**	37
	2.8	**The rationale for iron and folic acid vs. multiple micronutrient supplementation.**	38

2.9　Periconceptional iron and folic acid supplementation　　　41

2.10　Conclusion　　　42

LIST OF ABBREVIATIONS

BMI	Body mass index
CRP	C-reactive protein
FA	Folic acid
Hb	Hemoglobin
Hcy	Homocysteine
ID	Iron deficiency
IDA	Iron deficiency anemia
IFA	Iron and folic acid
IUGR	Intrauterine growth restriction
LBW	Low birth weight
MMN	Multiple micronutrient
NGO	Non-government organization
NTDs	Neural tube defects
RBCs	Red blood cells
RCT	Randomized controlled trial
TfR	Transferrin Receptor
US	United States
VS	Versus
WHO	World Health Organization

of IUGR include an increased risk of fetal, neonatal and infant death and impaired postnatal growth, immune function and intellectual development (10;11). Long-term consequences include an increased risk of adult chronic disease (cardiovascular disease and type 2 diabetes) (12;13).

Iron deficiency (ID): Broadly defined, ID is a condition in which there is a lack of cellular iron to tissues (6). ID represents a spectrum of mild to severe forms characterized by the presence or absence of physiological, biochemical, hematological and functional changes. Therefore, various definitions of ID have been formulated. The development of iron deficiency anemia (IDA) is commonly thought of as a progression of three successive stages: iron depletion, iron-deficient erythropoiesis (IDE), and IDA (7).

Iron-deficient erythropoiesis: Iron-deficient erythropoiesis (IDE) involves a decrease in transport iron resulting in low levels of serum ferritin and serum transferrin saturation and elevated levels of serum-transferrin receptor (TfR) and free erythrocyte protoporphyrin (FEP) (14). This stage is commonly referred to as ID without anemia. The iron supply required for full maturation of eyrthropoietic cells is markedly reduced; however, mature red blood cells stay unaffected (7). Hb concentrations usually remain within in the normal range, although they may decrease slightly. Unlike ID anemia, in which iron stores are totally absent, IDE can occur with normal or increased amounts of storage iron resulting from the impaired release of iron to the plasma from the storage iron compartment (6).

Iron deficiency anemia (IDA): IDA develops when the supply of transport iron decreases to the point where Hb synthesis is restricted (3). During this stage iron stores are exhausted, circulating levels of iron are declining and microcytic, hypochromic anemia is evident (15). A restricted supply of iron to the bone marrow causes a reduction in the concentration of Hb in the red blood cells and an observable decline in hematocrit and red cell indices.

Iron depletion: Iron depletion (ID) is characterized by a mobilization of storage iron (15). A fall in serum iron reflects the progressive reduction of storage iron in the liver; however, the supply of iron to the functional compartment remains uncompromised (9). Levels of transport iron and Hb remain normal. The absence of iron stores may not be associated with any adverse functional implications and should therefore only be regarded as a risk factor for the development of IDA (6).

Low birth weight (LBW): LBW babies are defined as weighing less than 2500 g at birth (7). Low birth weight affects large numbers of infants in developing countries (11). Premature delivery makes a major contribution and is frequently complicated by IUGR. In developing countries, IUGR is the predominant cause of LBW (11).

Multiple micronutrient supplement (MMN): In 1999, UNICEF, WHO, and the United Nations University recommended that MMN supplements should replace the existing IFA supplement (16). The composition of multiple micronutrient supplements for antenatal use included: vitamin A (800 µg), vitamin E (10 mg), vitamin D (5 µg), vitamin B1 (1.4 mg), vitamin B2 (1.4 mg), niacin (18 mg), vitamin B6 (1.9 mg), vitamin B12 (2.6 µg), folic acid (400 μg), vitamin C (70 mg), iron (30 mg), zinc (15 mg), copper (2 mg), selenium (65 μg), and iodine (150 μg).

Non-government organization (NGO): An NGO is a legally constituted organization that is created by private organizations or people with no participation or representation of any government.

Nulliparous: This term means never having given birth to a child.

Periconceptional period: The periconceptional period denotes the period from before conception to early pregnancy. There is no consensus in the literature on an exact time frame. The Institute of Medicine recommends that the periconceptional period be used to represent the period from 1 to 3 months prior to conception until 6 weeks of gestation (17).

Puberty: Puberty and adolescence are terms used to describe the period between childhood and adulthood (2). Puberty is defined as the period during which the reproductive system matures and ends when bone growth ceases (2). Cessation of bone growth occurs at 16 years for girls and at 17.5 years for boys (1).

Tranferrin Receptor: Soluble transferrin receptor (sTfR) is a critical iron binding protein in iron metabolism and has only recently been added to the available screening tests for ID (18). TfR reflects the degree of deficiency in functional iron after iron stores have been depleted. Inclusion of serum TfR in the determination of iron status is recommended because it can distinguish anemia of chronic disease from IDA in the presence of chronic infection or inflammation (7) . This noteworthy advantage contrasts with other biochemical tests for iron status, which are influenced by anemia of chronic disease. A major laboratory issue that remains unsolved is the lack of proper standardization for the sTfR assay: there are several commercial assays available for sTfR, but no common reference material (19).

1.0 INTRODUCTION

There is a growing interest in the area of maternal and child health that is advocating for a focus on the periconceptional period to improve iron and folate status among childbearing aged women before pregnancy. An association between periconceptional folate supplementation and reduction in neural tube defects (NTDs) is already well-established (20;21). For decades, public health programs have been promoting iron supplementation during pregnancy. Attention is now being given as to whether including periconceptional iron supplementation may complement iron supplementation during pregnancy to improve maternal and infant outcomes (22). In 2007, the National Strategy for Anemia Prevention and Control in Bangladesh included adolescents and newly married women as important target groups for iron and folic acid (IFA) supplementation programs (23). This thesis is aimed at providing evidence-based research to inform decision-making around periconceptional IFA programs in Bangladesh.

This thesis is comprised of two studies, a pilot study and a randomized controlled study. Both the pilot study and the RCT were conducted in a rural area in central Bangladesh. The studies were designed to expand our understanding of periconceptional IFA supplementation among women living in a rural area in Bangladesh. The pilot study examined individual factors associated with time to first pregnancy among ever-married women. The double-blinded randomized controlled trial (RCT) examined the effect of periconceptional iron supplementation on anemia and iron indicators before and during pregnancy. Both treatment groups received folic acid because periconceptional folic acid is recommended before a potential pregnancy to reduce the risk of neural tube defects. Secondary outcomes included side effects, adherence and plasma folate concentrations.

Results from these two studies are presented in three distinct but interrelated papers. The first paper (chapter 4) describes the results from the pilot study. The next two papers (chapters 5 and 6) report the findings from the RCT. The results from these three papers aim to provide impetus and directions for policy interventions to ameliorate anemia and iron deficiency (ID) among women of reproductive age in Bangladesh. This body of work is organized around two key themes:

i) Elucidation of individual factors associated with initiation of childbearing among women in rural Bangladesh. Information on age at marriage, contraceptive use and time to first pregnancy will inform the design and implementation of IFA supplementation programs to adolescents and newly married women.

ii) Examination of the iron and folate status of women in rural Bangladesh prior to IFA supplementation and after supplementation among non-pregnant and pregnant women. Information on iron and folate status prior to intervention will describe the magnitude of the problem. Results on the outcome of the trial will indicate whether or not the intervention was successful and will highlight challenges and issues for implementing periconceptional IFA supplementation programs

Following a review of the literature on iron and folate supplementation, the methods and results of these three papers are presented, followed by a discussion of the key findings and implications of this body of work to policy and future research directions.

2.0 LITERATURE REVIEW

2.1 Anemia: epidemiology, control and prevention

Anemia is one of the most common and widespread disorders in the world and affects one-quarter of the world's population (24). Anemia poses a serious threat to maternal and child health, contributing to low birth weight infants (LBW), a lowered resistance to infection, poor cognitive development and decreased work productivity (25). Young children and women of reproductive age have the highest rates of anemia (24). Among women of reproductive age, non-pregnant women, in numbers, are the most affected by anemia (~468 million); however, pregnant women have the highest prevalence rates (24). Global figures for the prevalence of anemia among non-pregnant and pregnant women are 35% and 51%, respectively (24).

The most common nutritional cause of anemia is ID (26). The consequences of ID include impaired cognitive performance, anemia, poor immune function and decreased work performance (27). The examination of an association between cognitive function and iron status has been extended to older children and adolescents. In a randomized controlled trial, adolescent girls with depleted iron stores who received iron supplements improved their scores on a test of memory and verbal learning compared with the placebo-treated group (28). Another large study in preadolescents and adolescents described an association between iron status and standardized mathematics scores (29). Those with IDA or ID without anemia were 2.3 and 2.4 times more likely to have low mathematics scores than those with no ID.

During pregnancy, the negative implications of anemia caused by ID alone or in combination with other factors, e.g., folate deficiency, vitamin A deficiency, and malaria, include increased risk of preterm delivery and infant low birth weight (30-33). There is some evidence to suggest severe anemia is associated with increased risk of maternal mortality (34;35). However, data were predominantly retrospective observations of maternal Hb concentrations at, or close to, delivery and subsequent mortality (34). Furthermore, the ID component of this relationship is unknown (35). Mechanisms by which IFA could increase maternal mortality needs to be elucidated. Rapid expansion of maternal blood volume and red cell mass during pregnancy and placental and foetal growth leave many women, even in developed countries, with low iron stores and tissue ID at parturition (36). The consequences of poor maternal iron status postpartum is increasingly being recognized as a non-benign condition and has been shown to be related to maternal fatigue, depression and ability to properly care and nurture offspring (37-39).

Global efforts to reduce the burden of anemia have largely been directed towards improving the iron status of children and pregnant women through diet diversification, food fortification and supplementation (40;41). Among women of reproductive age, industrialized nations have had greater success in reducing the prevalence of anemia compared to developing nations (42). Industrialized nations have used public health strategies to reduce anemia including education, iron fortification and therapeutic approaches (43;44). The most sustainable intervention for maintaining adequate iron status is a food-based dietary approach that relies on sustained ingestion of adequate amounts of bioavailable iron from food (45). However, a food-based dietary approach is challenging because it is difficult to change food habits and preparation practices and iron-rich foods are costly to poor populations (46). Therefore a preferred approach to preventing IDA in the general population is iron fortification, which ensures an adequate amount of bioavailable iron in the food supply (42). Iron fortification of staple foods and commonly used condiments in combination with iron supplementation are more practical solutions (45). Iron fortification has been used to enhance iron intake in many developed countries for more than 50 years, but it has only been in the last decade that this strategy has been applied on a large scale to other parts of the world (47). There are several issues that remain to be addressed, such as the concern that people in the target population may not consume enough of the fortified food and questions regarding who will bear the cost of fortification and provide regulatory monitoring to ensure quality assurance (42). Experience from existing fortification programs indicate that fortification is financially feasible as long as the cost is shouldered by the consumer (42). Further research is needed to evaluate whether poor people in developing countries consume sufficient quantities and are able to afford the additional cost of the fortified food item.

In developing countries, the most common strategy to control and treat anemia in pregnant women thus far, has been through supplementation (42). The provision of iron supplements to pregnant women is one of the most widely practiced public health measures (34). Recognizing that folate is the second most common nutritional cause of anemia and that folate nutrition plays an important role in human reproduction (48;49), formulations of supplements to pregnant women have commonly included iron and folic acid (50).

2.2 Prevention and control of anemia in developing countries

The prevention and control of anemia and ID in developing countries is much more challenging than in industrialized nations (42). The magnitude of the problem is far greater and the availability of resources is much more limited. In the industrialized world, estimates suggest that

≥30% of pregnant women will have depleted iron stores by the end of pregnancy, and in some population groups (e.g., adolescents) depleted iron stores could occur in ≥80% of the population (25;51). While a large proportion of pregnant women in the industrialized world still begin pregnancy with low or completely depleted iron stores, inadequate iron nutrition is mainly a problem in developing countries (52).

In developing countries, IDA in pregnancy is highly prevalent (53). It has been estimated that 47% of pregnant women in Africa, 39% of pregnant women in Latin America, 80% of pregnant women in Southeast Asia, 65% of pregnant women in the eastern Mediterranean, and 40% of pregnant women in the West Pacific are anemic (54). Sub-clinical ID is nearly as widespread as IDA (43). Risk of IDA is particularly high in women who begin gestation with depleted or low body iron stores, a situation common in Africa and most Third World countries (25;55). Iron requirements during pregnancy are not easily satisfied by dietary intakes, which generally provide poor iron bioavailability (56).

2.3 Risk factors associated with adolescent childbearing

Adolescents are one of the groups most at risk for developing anemia and ID during pregnancy (57-59). Women encounter high iron requirements to meet the demands of the adolescent growth spurt and the onset of menstruation (60). Iron is essential for skeletal growth and ID may be a limiting factor for growth during adolescence (60). Early marriage, a cultural norm in South Asian countries, often leads to childbearing during the adolescent years (61). Pregnancy and motherhood frequently occurs before adolescents are fully developed physically, exposing mother and child to acute health risks during pregnancy and childbirth (62).

2.3.1 Maternal outcomes

Adolescent pregnancies are associated with increased risk of maternal death (63), attributed to poor socioeconomic status, gynecological immaturity and growth, and poor nutritional status of the mother. It is well documented that growth velocity during adolescence is slower in undernourished populations, giving rise to cephaelopelvic disproportion in adolescents who become pregnant, which is related to increased maternal and foetal mortality (64). The birth canal does not reach its mature size until several years after growth in height has ceased by the age of 18 years (65). As a result, cephalopelvic disproportion (CPD) is the commonest problem encountered during labour in teenage pregnancies, as pelvis architecture incompletely formed and not mature enough for delivery (65). Women who are stunted are more likely to experience obstructed labour and a greater risk of dying in childbirth (66). Adolescent girls have a 2–5 times greater risk of mortality than do other women of reproductive age (67). In countries with poor general health conditions and inadequate healthcare services the risks involved with adolescent pregnancy are even more severe (68).

Recent attention has been raised towards improving the iron status of adolescents, especially in South Asia countries (58). The promotion of optimal nutrition in girls during childhood is being proposed as a strategy for improving female nutrition by building nutritional reserves needed during periods of increased nutritional demand, including the adolescent growth spurt, pregnancy, and lactation (22;58;69). Concern for the health of young mothers and their infants has led to suggestions that adolescence may be an ideal time to optimize iron status and prevent ID during pregnancy (58).

2.3.2 Infant outcomes

Children born to adolescent mothers are more likely to be of poor health and have a higher likelihood of infant mortality (35). In comprehensive study in developing countries, Nestle and Rutstein (70) evaluated data from 46 national surveys in 36 developing countries for mothers aged 15-49 years. Women with a low BMI had the poorest outcomes for neonatal mortality, infant mortality, size at birth and birth weight compared to women with normal or high BMI (70). Women with low BMI were more likely to have an infant that was smaller or of lower birth weight than infants born to women with either normal or high BMI (70). Impaired nutrient supply to fetus results in inappropriate in utero growth, reduced size at birth and increased risk of mortality and morbidity (71). In girls who are still growing at the time of conception, adolescent pregnancy is associated with increased risk of spontaneous miscarriage, prematurity and low birth weight (71). The Camden study examined continued growth among adolescents who became pregnant (72). During pregnancy, continued maternal growth was associated with larger maternal weight gain, increased body fat stores and greater postpartum weight retention (72). Despite these changes which could be thought to be associated with increased fetal size, growing pregnant women have infants with birth weights reduced by 150 to 200 g compared with non-growing pregnant women (72). Competition between the mother and fetus for nutrients was suggested by marked reductions in placental blood flow on a Doppler ultrasound and reduced micronutrients in the fetus from the still-growing mother (73). Studies of still growing pregnant sheep suggest that incomplete maternal growth is an independent risk factor for LBW delivery because early in gestation the physiological changes associated with ongoing maternal growth impede placentation, and permanently restrict fetal growth (71).

Epidemiological studies provide evidence that adolescents are at high risk giving birth to LBW (<2500 g) (63) and that LBW, even within the normal range, is a risk factor in later life for development of obesity, stroke, diabetes, immune dysfunction and cardiovascular disease (12;13). Studies that include variables known to affect neonatal outcomes such as pre-pregnant BMI, smoking and SES suggest that infant size is more related to maternal size than to maternal age (74). In the US, the highest rate of adolescent pregnancy in the developed world, offspring of adolescent mothers are reported as having poorer cognitive development, lower educational attainment, more frequent criminal activity and a higher risk of abuse, neglect and behavioural problems during childhood (75).

2.4 Iron

With the exception of certain members of the bacterial genera, iron is an essential nutrient for all living organisms. Iron is a versatile and highly reactive group-VIII transition metal with electrons distributed throughout five 3d orbitals (76). Depending on the chemical environment iron can exist in several oxidation states (between -2 and +6). At physiological oxygen concentrations iron exists in its stable ferric (Fe^{3+}) state for most of its biological complexes. Ferrous (Fe^{2+}) iron is used in transmembrane transport of iron, deposition of iron in the storage protein and synthesis of heme (77). The only stable iron states in the aqueous environment of the human body and in food are ferric and ferrous iron. The human body contains 2 to 4 grams of elemental iron, most of which is in the Hb of erythrocytes (78). Over 65% of body iron is present in the Hb, up to 10% is found in myoglobin and approximately 1% to 5% is present as part of enzymes (79).

Iron is vital for metabolic processes such as oxygen transport, DNA synthesis and electron transport (80). Tissue oxygenation is iron's key function. Oxygen is bound to an iron-containing porphyrin ring, either as part of the prosthetic group of Hb within erythrocytes, or as part of myoglobin located within the cytoplasm of muscle cells (80).

2.4.1 Iron metabolism

Iron absorption occurs in the proximal duodenum and involves a sequence of events: (a) reduction; (b) apical uptake; (c) intracellular storage or trafficking and; (d) basolateral release (81). Clinical disorders that affect iron absorption include malabsorption syndromes such as steatorrhea and tropical sprue (76).

(a) Reduction: Most inorganic iron in the diet is in the oxidized or ferric form (81). Before iron can be taken up by the intestinal epithelial cells or enterocytes, iron must first be reduced from its ferric to ferrous form in the luminal brush border of the enterocyte. Ferrous iron is more readily absorbed than ferric iron due to higher solubility in the proximal small intestine. Iron reduction is facilitated by the acidic milieu of the gastric content and the meal composition (82).

(b) Apical uptake: In order to reach the plasma, iron must pass from the gut through the apical (lumenal) and basolateral (serosal) membranes of the enterocyte (82). Absorptive cells located in the crypts of the duodenum are organized as finger-like villous structures to increase surface area. Beginning as stem cells, these absorptive cells proliferate and migrate out of the crypt and up to the villus over a period of several days (83). During migration the cells differentiate and perform their functions (84). During the intestinal phase of digestion iron is present in the lumen as either heme or non-heme iron. The pathway by which heme iron is absorbed is less well defined than that of inorganic iron (82). A specific duodenal receptor/transporter for heme has not yet been elucidated in humans (81). Heme iron is released from proteins such as Hb and myoglobin in the lumen of the stomach and small intestine (82). While the chemical form of the resulting „free" heme has not been well defined, it is likely stabilized by various dietary constituents, including Hb degradation products. Luminal absorption of heme does not require binding proteins because heme iron is soluble in an alkaline environment. After binding to its receptor, heme iron is absorbed intact by the intestinal enterocytes (8). Iron from heme is not released prior to its cellular uptake, making heme iron less susceptible than inorganic heme to variations in dietary composition (85). The percent iron absorption from heme iron is five-to-ten fold higher than that from non-heme iron. Most studies have shown that ID is able to stimulate the absorption of both heme iron and inorganic iron (85).

(c) Intracellular storage or trafficking: Once iron has been absorbed by enterocytes it is bound by, as of yet unidentified, chaperones (80). Inside the absorptive enterocyte, iron can either be stored as ferritin or transferred across the basolateral membrane into the circulation where it will be bind to apoferritin (86). Proteins related to iron metabolism on the basolateral membrane of the precursor and mature enterocyte either sense body iron stores or facilitate regulated iron transport into the plasma. These proteins include the transferrin receptor-hereditary hemochromatosis protein (HFE) complex, the basolateral iron transporter and the ceruloplasmin homologue, hephaestin (84). Iron that remains in the form of ferritin as the enterocyte completes it life cycle will be sloughed off with the senescent cell and exit the body through the gastrointestinal tract. This maturation process takes approximately three to five days (87).

(d) Basolateral release: The pathways by which inorganic and heme iron are taken up from the intestinal lumen by the enterocytes vary; however, it has been proposed that their basolateral export from enterocytes, i.e. the step involving hepaestin and IREG1, is common to iron from both sources. The basolateral membrane mediates the transfer of iron from the intestinal epithelial cells to the rest of the body (84). Once inside the epithelial cell heme is either split into ferrous iron and bilirubin by heme oxygenase, or transported as the intact porphyrin ring (85). The released ferrous iron likely enters the pool of iron in the enterocyte and exits the enterocyte via a pathway common to inorganic iron (88). If required by the body, iron rapidly moves across the basolateral membrane and into the circulation. The major molecule that carries iron across the basolateral membrane is ferroportin (also known as IREG1, MTP1) (82). A multicopper ferroxidase, hephaestin, acts in a way, as of yet unknown, to facilitate basolateral iron transport (76). Hephaestin may serve to oxidize iron in order to allow binding of iron to the plasma iron carrier, transferrin (89). Once iron transverses the basolateral membrane it is bound to transferrin.

When intracellular iron exceeds cellular requirements, excess iron is kept in storage. All cells are capable of storing iron; however, principal storage sites in humans are the liver, spleen and bone marrow (77). The concentration of storage iron in the body varies by gender and iron status. Iron is stored in the form of ferritin or hemosiderin. Ferritin is comprised of 24 similar polypeptide subunits that form a cage isolating iron from the cellular milieu. Hemosiderin, is an

LIST OF DEFINITIONS

Adolescence: The end of adolescence (~19 years) is defined less clearly than puberty and is characterized by a mixture of physical, psychological, social and mental measures (1). Adolescence is comprised of physiological, psychological, and social constructs (2). Chronologists and biologists have not been able to precisely define when adolescence ends (2). The Dietary Reference Intakes for iron define adolescence as 14 to 18 years of age (3). The World Health Organization (WHO) defines adolescence as 10-19 years of age (4).

Anemia: Anemia is defined as a decrease in the concentration of circulating red blood cells or in the Hb concentration causing impaired capacity to transport oxygen (5). Anemia has multiple precipitating factors that can occur in isolation but more frequently co-exist. These precipitating factors include genetic factors, such as hemoglobinopathies; infections (i.e. malaria, or intestinal helminthes) and nutritional deficiencies, such as iron folate, vitamin A and vitamin B12 (6).

Body mass index: Body mass index (BMI) is calculated from dividing weight by the square of height (7). In adults BMI is a reliable and valid indicator of obesity at the population level. BMI correlates well with percentage of body fat and is relatively unbiased by height (7).

Erythrocyte folate: Erythrocytes incorporate folate during formation in the bone marrow (7). The lifespan of the erythrocyte cell is ~120 days; therefore, erythrocyte folate concentrations are a relatively long term marker of folate status. Erythrocyte folate concentrations correlate well with liver folate levels; thus representing folate stores (7).

Ferritin: Serum and erythrocyte ferritin concentrations reflect the level of storage iron (8). Serum measurements are simpler and are the more common of the two tests (9). Having been found to be directly proportional to the abundance of storage iron in normal subjects, serum fferritin concentration is used as a sensitive and specific index for ID (3). When used in combination with the measurement of Hb, serum ferritin distinguishes between the anemias of chronic disease and ID (7). A low serum ferritin concentration is usually interpreted as depleted iron stores, but does not necessarily indicate systemic ID. When iron stores have been completely exhausted the concentration of serum ferritin no longer reflects the severity of ID (6).

Folate deficiency: The initial stage of folate deficiency results from a period of negative folate balance (7). If negative folate balance persists, folate depletion occurs, which is characterized by declining liver stores and a fall in erythrocyte folate concentrations. At this stage of folate depletion, there is no evidence of clinical impairment (7). With further deprivation, biochemical function is impaired, a stage often referred to as folate-deficient erythropoiesis, or sub clinical deficiency (7). The final stage of folate depletion is folate deficiency anemia; this stage is characterized by the macro-ovalocytic erythrocytes and low Hb levels (7).

Hemoglobin (Hb): Hb concentration measures the presence of anemia (7;9) and is the most widely used screening tool for ID. However, Hb determination has serious limitations when relied upon as the only laboratory measurement because of its low specificity and sensitivity (7).

Intrauterine growth restriction (IUGR): IUGR is defined as a birth weight below the 10th percentile for gestational age based on a standard population (10;11). Short-term consequences ill-defined water-soluble degradation product of ferritin that appears to result from incomplete lysomal processing (77). The type of iron stored in hemosiderin is less chemically reactive than what is found in ferritin and potentially less available for mobilization (76).

The liver contains about 60% of the ferritin in the body with the remaining amount present in muscle tissues and cells of the reticuloenthelial system. Macrophages act as a storage depot for iron recovered from effete erythrocytes or from medicinal forms of iron administered by injection. Their storage capacity is evident when tissues from patients with transfusional iron overload are stained for iron; large amounts of iron accumulate in macrophages before deposition in parenchymal cells becomes apparent (89).

2.4.2   Iron requirements among women of reproductive age

Iron requirements are high during periods of rapid growth such as the first years of life, adolescence and pregnancy (90). ID can arise from several risk factors, alone or in combination. Examples from the range of possible risk factors include: a) inadequate iron supply, b) increased iron requirements imposed by growth and c) increased iron losses (**Table** 2.4.2). Adolescence is the second most critical period of physical growth in the life cycle (60). During adolescence iron requirements nearly double in both boys and girls as a result of the expansion of the total blood volume and the increase in lean body mass (60). Estimates of physiological iron requirements during the adolescent period have been computed using a factorial method of iron components (basal losses, menstrual losses, and accretion) (3). Preadolescent levels of overall iron requirements (0.7– 0.9 mg Fe/d) increase to as much as 2.2 mg Fe/d (91). Female adolescents require an additional amount of iron to account for iron losses during menses. Menstrual losses may increase daily requirements to as much as 2.1 mg/d in girls at the 75th percentile of blood loss (60). Among 14 year old girls, median iron requirements can be 30% higher than for their mothers (92). Iron requirements may increase further in heavily menstruating young women.

During pregnancy iron requirements rise significantly due to increased red cell mass, the expansion of plasma volume and growth of the fetal-placental unit (56). The additional iron requirement for pregnancy (3-4 mg/d) is substantial and it is estimated that fewer than 50% of women have adequate iron stores to meet this additional need (93). Furthermore, iron requirements are not distributed equally over the duration of pregnancy. Requirements are low in the first trimester (due to the absence of menstrual iron losses and the negligible needs of fetus) but rise to between 4 and 6 mg in the second and third trimesters, respectively (56). During the last 6 to 8 weeks of pregnancy requirements may reach as much as 10 mg/d (9).

By the end of pregnancy, approximately 1200 mg of iron is required, either from body iron stores or from the diet (90). The average requirement for a menstruating woman for the same period of time is roughly 400 mg. In order to accommodate this increased requirement of 800 mg and avoid a negative iron balance the average woman must absorb 500 mg (2 mg/d) more iron than she required while menstruating (90). In most cases, dietary intakes alone are insufficient to meet the requirements of pregnancy, especially in the latter part of pregnancy (90). It is, therefore, estimated that a female needs 500 mg of stored iron to cover iron requirements during pregnancy (9). A woman who routinely eats a diet high in bioavailable iron and enters pregnancy with sufficient iron stores will likely meet her requirements (56). However, a higher amount of stored iron is needed when the diet is less than optimal (9).

Table 2.4.2: Main factors that negatively influence iron balance

Birth	Infancy	Childhood and Adolescence
Before birth Maternal iron deficiency Intrauterine growth retardation **At birth** Low body iron stores at birth Early onset of postnatal erythropoiesis Rapid postnatal catch-up growth Low birth weight Premature birth Fetal-maternal hemorrhage Perinatal hemorrhage Twin-to-twin transfusion Umbilical cord preclamping Phlebotomy losses Restrictive RBC transfusion practice Recombinant erythropoietin administration (preterm infants)	**0-6 months** Low/depleted body iron stores Rapid weight gain Blood loss due to frequent sampling Blood loss due to cow milk feeding **6-12 months** Low/depleted iron stores Rapid weight gain Blood loss due to cow milk feeding Low dietary iron supply Low dietary iron availability Prolonged exclusive breastfeeding Frequent infections	Antacid therapy Low dietary iron supply Low dietary iron availability Intense physical activity Adolescent pregnancy Loss or dysfunction of absorptive enterocytes Bowel resection Celiac disease Intrinsic enterocyte defects Gastrointestinal blood loss: epistaxis, varices, gastritis, ulcer, tumor, meckel"s diverticulum, parasitosis, vascular malformations, inflammatory bowel disease, diverticulosis, hemorrhoids, menorrhagia, cancer, chronic infection, pulmonary hemosiderosis, trauma, excessive phlebotomy, large vascular malformations

2.4.3 Dietary sources of iron

A normal diet contains approximately 13-18 mg of iron per day, of which only 1 mg of iron per day is needed in healthy persons to replace basal iron losses (87). While many foods are good sources of iron, some are limited by the bioavailability of iron. Iron-rich foods include cocoa, liver, kidney, dried fish, shell-fish, sesame seed, soy flour and pulses (94). Foods with low-iron content include milk, cheese, sugar, sweets, jams, and unfortified milled cereals.

There are two forms of iron in the diet – inorganic iron and heme iron. Heme iron is present in the Hb and myoglobin of animal tissues and is thus mainly associated with meat, poultry and fish intake (95). In a single meal 5% to 35% of heme iron is absorbed (85). Studies using radiolabelled heme or Hb have established that the intestinal absorption of heme is far more efficient than inorganic iron (8). Heme iron is well absorbed regardless of meal composition with the exception of meat and calcium. Meat has been shown to enhance heme iron absorption (96). Calcium is the only dietary factor known to negatively influence the absorption of heme iron and does so to the same extent that it influences non-heme iron (97).

Inorganic iron, predominantly found in components of plant origin, is the most prevalent form of dietary iron (98). Inorganic iron accounts for 80–90% of the iron in a standard diet (76). Non-heme iron is generally poorly absorbed and greatly influenced by enhancing or inhibiting substances (94). Meat, fish amino acids and organic acids (i.e. ascorbic acid, lactic acid, citric acid and malic acid) promote non-heme iron absorption (98;99). Phenols, calcium and phytates which are present in cereals and legumes, impair non-heme iron absorption (94). Phenolic compounds, which bear catechol or galloyl groups, have iron-binding properties (94). Tea, coffee, cocoa, red wine, many vegetables (such as spinach), grains, herbs and spices (such as oregano and cinnamon) contain phenolic compounds. Vitamin A may be capable of preventing the inhibiting effect of polyphenols on iron absorption (94). Phytates are a storage form of phosphates and minerals in cereals, seeds, nuts, vegetables and fruit. Bran, oats and fiber-rich foods are rich in phytates. The effect of phytates is counteracted by ascorbic acid, meat, fish and poultry (94).

2.4.4 Assessment of iron status

The most important clinical clue of moderate to severe chronic ID in adults is chronic fatigue (15). Other features include: pallor of the skin and of the conjunctiva, stomatitis, ice eating (pagophagia), leg cramping, koilonychia, glossitis, gastric atrophy and dysphagia. It is also possible that some individuals with ID may not experience any symptoms (76). Since clinical signs of anemia are not specific, it is recommended that biochemical tests be used to determine ID and its magnitude (100).

Among the wide variety of laboratory methods that are available to assess iron status (i.e. hematocrit, Hb, mean cell volume, erythrocyte mean index, free erythrocyte protoporphyrin, serum iron, total iron-binding capacity, serum transferrin, transferrin saturation, serum ferritin and serum transferrin receptor) there is no one single test that is ideal. Diminished stainable iron in a bone marrow aspirate is generally accepted to be the reference standard for iron status (101). However, the method is invasive, costly and subject to variable interpretation.

Rather than using a single measurement, a valid assessment of iron status is best characterized by multiple indices (14). Presently, there is no consensus on the best definition of ID using multiple measures. Features of the more commonly accepted diagnostic indices are summarized in **Table 2.4.4**. For a detailed review see Gibson (7).

2.4.4.1 Hemoglobin

Hb measures the presence of anemia and is the most widely used screening tool for ID. Hb determination has serious limitations when relied upon as the only laboratory measurement because of its low specificity and sensitivity (15). When used alone Hb concentration does not distinguish between anemia due to ID and that due to infection (e.g., malaria, HIV), other micronutrient deficiencies (e.g., folate, vitamin B12, vitamin A) or other disease states (e.g. sickle cell disease, thalassemia). Furthermore, the wide range of values in normal subjects means that Hb values overlap considerably between normal and IDA individuals (9).

Table 2.4.4: Selected Biochemical indices for measuring iron status

Indicator	Measurement	Advantages and Disadvantages	Factors that Affect Measurement
Hemoglobin (Hb)	Decreased concentration of Hb measures presence of anemia; most widely used test for IDA	**Advantages** Inexpensive; universally available **Disadvantages** Low sensitivity; low specificity	Diurnal variation, age, sex, race, pregnancy, high altitudes, other micronutrient deficiencies, parasitic infections, disease states
Hematocrit	Ratio of the volume of packed red blood cells to the total blood volume; indicator of the concentration of RBCs in the blood and impaired Hb formation; in presence of anemia decrease in red blood cells is observed	**Advantages** Inexpensive; requires a small sample volume; relatively fast analysis **Disadvantages** Sensitive to changes in plasma volume, as well as red cell volume; difficult to standardize because it is a calculated parameter	Measurement errors (poorly packed iron-deficient cells, improper mixing of blood because of intermittent blood flow, excessive anticoagulant in collection tube); elevated white blood cell counts; vitamin B12 deficiency, bleeding, kidney disease, cirrhosis of the liver, and malignancies; pregnancy.
Mean cell volume (MCV)	Average volume of a red cell; calculated by dividing hematocrit (volume fraction) by red blood cell count (10^2/L)	**Advantages** Inexpensive; fairly specific indicator of iron deficiency once thalassemia and the anemia of chronic disease have been excluded	Chronic inflammation, certain hemoglobinopathies, lead poisoning, age, race
Serum iron	In fasting state serum iron levels reflect transit iron going from reticulo-endothethial system to the bone marrow	**Advantages** Sensitive to the stage of mild iron deficiency **Disadvantages** Wide diurnal variations; low specificity	Diurnal variation, age, sex, inflammation, chronic neoplastic diseases, blood loss or donation, pregnancy, with chronic infections, shock, pyrexia, rheumatoid arthritis and malignancy.
Ferritin	Serum or plasma iron concentration reflects total amount of storage iron.	**Advantages** Reliable and sensitive parameter for iron stores in healthy subjects; high specificity for iron deficiency **Disadvantages** Does not indicate the severity of the iron deficiency due to higher assay variability; acute phase reactant.	Diurnal effect is minimal, age, sex, race, inflammatory diseases, infections, certain neoplastic diseases and liver disorders.
Serum transferrin receptor (sTfR)	An increase in serum receptor levels is seen in patients with iron deficient erythropoiesis or iron deficiency anemia	**Advantages** Remains normal in patients with acute or chronic inflammation or liver disease; effective in distinguishing iron deficiency anemia from anemia of chronic disease **Disadvantages** Lack of standardization for assay and reference values. Expensive assay cost.	Hematologic disorders associated with expansion of erythroid marrow

Affected by diurnal variations; Hb values in the evening tend to be lower than values in the morning by up to 10 g/L (7). It is essential to interpret Hb concentration according to age-specific and sex-specific reference standards (102).

2.4.4.2 Ferritin

Serum and erythrocyte ferritin concentrations reflect the level of storage iron (8). Serum measurements are simpler and are the more common of the two tests (6). Having been found to be directly proportional to the abundance of storage iron in normal subjects, serum ferritin concentration is used as a sensitive and specific index for ID. When used in combination with the measurement of Hb, serum ferritin distinguishes between the anemias of chronic disease and ID (15).

A low serum ferritin concentration is usually interpreted as depleted iron stores, but does not necessarily indicate systemic ID. Adequate iron for erythropoiesis can be maintained even in the presence of low stores, as occurs in frequent blood donors (14). When iron stores have been completely exhausted the concentration of serum ferritin no longer reflects the severity of ID.

The absence of iron stores may not be associated with any adverse functional implications and should therefore only be regarded as a risk factor for the development of IDA (9). The most important limitation of ferritin is its acute phase response, which can mask an otherwise iron-depletion state in clinical conditions such as infection, inflammation, and malignancy (9). To overcome this limitation, simultaneous measurement of a biomarker of the acute-phase response such as C-reactive protein and screening for the presence of malaria parasites should be conducted (9). The cut-off value for serum ferritin indicating depleted iron stores that is most commonly used is 12 µg/L (6;25).

2.4.4.3 Tranferrin Receptor

Soluble transferrin receptor (sTfR), a critical iron binding protein in iron metabolism, has only recently been added to the available screening tests for ID (19). The transferrin receptor (TfR) reflects the degree of deficiency in functional iron after iron stores have been depleted (19). Inclusion of serum TfR in the determination of iron status is recommended because it can distinguish anemia of chronic disease from IDA in the presence of chronic infection or inflammation (9). This noteworthy advantage contrasts with other biochemical tests for iron status, which are influenced by anemia of chronic disease.

It should be emphasized that the sTfR cannot be used in isolation of other laboratory measurements to identify iron deficiency anemia (IDA) in anemic patients, because it is also elevated in hematologic disorders associated with expansion of the erythroid marrow (18). Certain conditions affecting erythropoiesis such as hematological disorders (e.g., sickle cell anemia, autoimmune hemolytic anemia, thalassemia) and nutritional deficiencies other than iron (e.g., folate, vitamin B12) may confound the diagnosis of ID since they have been demonstrated to raise sTfR concentration (18). Hemolysis associated with malaria may elevate sTfR concentration and confuse the detection of ID, although the magnitude of this effect remains unknown.

A major laboratory issue that remains unsolved is the lack of proper standardization for the sTfR assay: there are several commercial assays available for sTfR, but no common reference material

(103). Over the past decade, a number of laboratories have developed different assays for measuring sTfR concentration and have explored its normal range. The normal range for sTfR reported in the literature varies considerably (19). To date, there are no standards for measuring sTfR. The ratio of serum transferrin receptor (sTfR) to serum ferritin (R/F ratio) has been shown to perform well in estimating body iron stores (104). Further research is needed regarding age appropriate cut-offs and the standardization of laboratory techniques such as the use of anticoagulant, blood collection methods, time delay between blood collection and centrifugation, incubation time, and the extent to which samples have to be diluted (103).

2.5 Folate

The term folic acid can designate a specific compound, pteroylglutamic acid (PGA), but is more commonly used as a general term for a class of related compounds (also called folates) with similar nutritional activity (105). Folate is essential for cell division and homeostasis; functioning as a coenzyme in single-carbon transfers in the metabolism of nucleic and amino acids (3). Folates only function as coenzymes in polyglutamate form; therefore, the folate monoglutamate forms in the blood must be reduced by folylpolyglutamate synthase and then resynthesized to the polyglutamate form (7). Biochemical reactions involving folate include phases of amino acid metabolism, purine and pyrimidine sythesthesis and the formation of the methylating agent, *S*-adenosylmethionine (SAM) (106).

Folic acid is the most oxidized and stable form of folate (3). Folic acid rarely occurs in food but is used in vitamin supplements and fortified food products.

Folic acid consists of a *p*-aminobenzoic acid molecule connected at one end to a pteridine ring and at the other end to one glutamic acid molecule. Pteroylpolyglutamates, also commonly referred to as food folates, contain a peptide linkage of one to six additional glutamate molecules joined to the γ-carboxyl of glutamate.

2.5.1 Folate metabolism

Folate absorption is an active process that primarily takes place in the small intestine. Food folates are hydrolyzed to monoglutamate forms in the gut (7). The molecule that cleaves the food folates is called γ-glutamylhydolase; also referred to as folate conjugase (3). The monoglutamate form of folate is transported across the proximal small intestine via an active and saturable pH-dependent process; however passive diffusion can occur by a non-saturable mechanism when pharmacological doses are consumed (**Figure 2.5.1**).

Most of the monoglutamates that are absorbed by the mucosal cells are transported to the liver and are metabolized to polyglutamate derivatives by the enzyme folylpolyglutamate synthetase. These derivatives can be retained in the liver or released into the blood or bile. Average folate concentrations in the liver of an adult human are estimated to be 11 mg, approximately half of total body folate (3). Polyglutamate derivatives in the liver that are secreted into the bile are first converted to 5-methyltetrahydrofolate, which are then reabsorbed via the enterohepatic circulation.

Figure 2.5.1: Overview of folate metabolism.

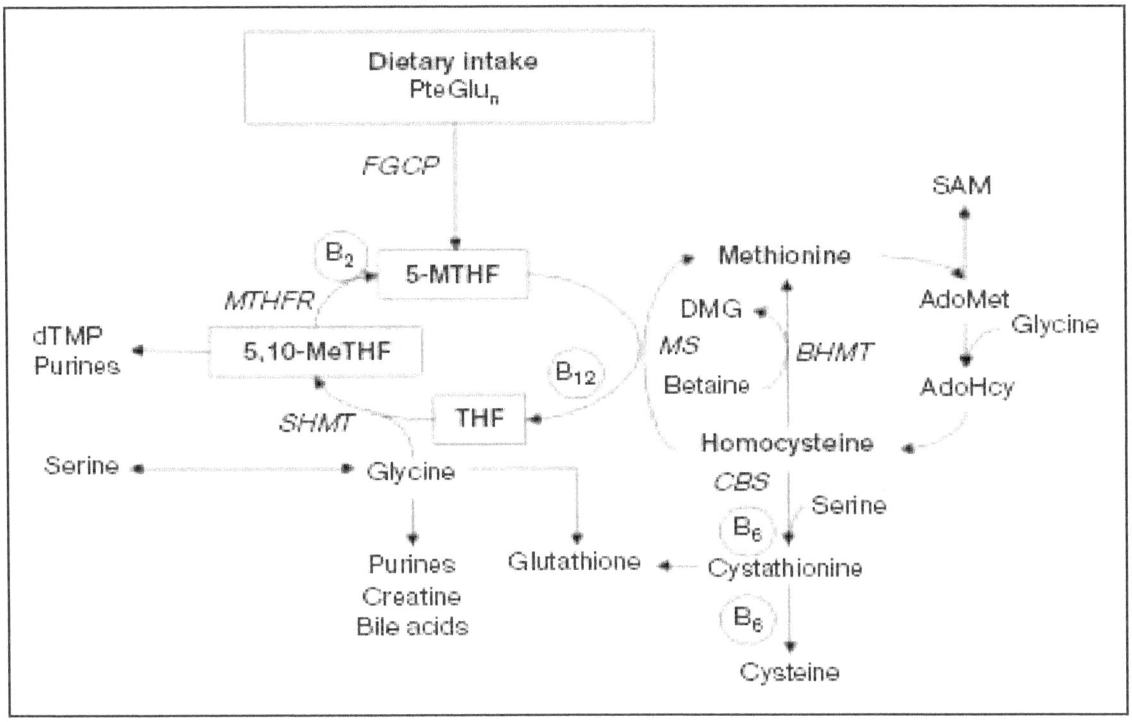

Adapted from Melse-Boostra et al. (107).

In the one-carbon cycle, the central folate acceptor is a polyglutamyl form of tetrahydrofolate (THF) (106). The first step in the cycle involving the 3-carbon of serine is the conversion of THF to 5, 10-methylene-THF. A one-carbon unit is transferred from serine to THF to form 5, 10-methylene-THF and glycine. A portion of the 5, 10-methylenetetrahydrofolate that is produced undergoes irreversible enzymatic reduction to the methyl oxidation state (as 5-methyl-THF) by methylene tetrahydrofolate reductase (MTHFR). The N-5 methyl group of 5-methyl-THF can only be used metabolically for transfer to homocysteine, which results in the (re)generation of methionine. MTHFR serves a key role in one-carbon metabolism by converting methylene-THF to 5-methyl-THF, thus irreversibly directing this one-carbon group to methylation of homocysteine synthesis.

2.5.2 Folate requirements among women of reproductive age

Folate requirements were estimated using erythrocyte folate in combination with plasma homocysteine and folate concentrations. The Recommended Dietary Allowance (RDA) for folate for both men and women is 400 µg/day of dietary folate equivalents (DFEs). DFEs adjust for the 50 percent lower availability of food folate compared to folic acid from fortified food or as a supplement. To reduce the risk of NTDs for women capable for becoming pregnant, 400 µg of folic acid is recommended daily from fortified foods, supplements or both, in addition to consuming food folate from a varied diet.

There are several factors that affect folate requirement; these include: the bioavailability of folic acid and food folate, nutrient-nutrient interactions, interactions with other food components, smoking, folate-drug interactions and genetic variations. The bioavailability of folate ranges from about 100 percent for folic acid supplements consumed on an empty stomach to approximately 50 percent for food folate (3). Relatively little is known regarding nutritional interactions that affect folate bioavailability. Concern has been expressed regarding a proposed mutually inhibitory effect of zinc and folate (108).

During pregnancy, the acceleration in cell division causes an increase in single-carbon transfer reactions, leading to substantially higher folate requirements. Cells multiply for uterine enlargement, placental development, expansion of maternal erythrocyte number and fetal growth. Moreover, folate is transferred to the fetus. For pregnant women, the maintenance of erythrocyte folate was used to indicate folate adequacy. When erythrocyte folate measurements were not available, serum folate concentrations were used while recognizing that hemodilution causes a normal reduction in serum folate concentration during gestation. Data from a series of population studies indicated that 600 μg/day of DFEs is adequate to maintain normal folate status in groups of pregnant women (3).

2.5.3 Dietary sources of folate

Folates are widely distributed in foods such as liver, yeast, leafy vegetables, fruits, pulses and nuts (107). Food folates exist primarily as pteroylpolyglutamates. The nutritional activity of polyglutamates remains intact as long as the essential subunit structure of PGA is not broken. Heat, air and ultraviolet light cleave PGA, rendering it inactive. Folate may also be lost during the food preparation process because of leaching from the food into cooking water. The presence in foods of antioxidants (ascorbic acid) and reduced thiols protects folate against oxidant instability; whereas the exposure to the peptic acid of the stomach increases folate instability (109).

In most industrialized countries, ready-to-eat cereals represent the most significant source of food folate (107). An increasing trend to fortify cereal grains with folate has led to increased folate intakes in many countries. Fortification was introduced in the United States and Canada in 1998. The United States enriched cereal grains at a level of 1.4 mg/kg grain (110); whereas, Canada selected a level of 1.5 mg/kg for both wheat flour and cornmeal (111).

2.5.4 Assessment of folate status

Folate deficiency is usually suspected because of the presence of unexplained anemia or macrocytosis. Folate deficiency can be caused from inadequate intake, increased demands, and malabsorption and from drugs with anti-folate activity. Epidemiological studies have demonstrated an association between inadequate folate status and the risk of vascular disease, certain cancers and the occurrence of a neural tube defect in an infant should pregnancy occur (108;112). Folate status is commonly assessed using biochemical tests that measure folate levels in serum and erythrocytes (7). Homocysteine in serum or plasma is increasingly being used as a functional test of folate deficiency (7).

2.5.4.1 Erythrocyte folate

The primary indicator for determining folate adequacy is erythrocyte folate. Erythrocyte folate reflects tissue folate stores. Folate is taken up by the developing erythrocyte in the bone marrow, which is characterized by a 120-day lifespan. Erythrocyte folate concentration does not reflect recent or transient changes in dietary folate intake. Based on several experiments, a value of 305 nmol/L (140 ng/mL) of folate is commonly used as the threshold for adequate folate status. Determination of red blood cell (RBC) folate levels is advocated as a measure of folate tissue stores.

2.5.4.2 Serum folate

Approximately two-thirds of folate in the serum is bound to protein (7). The main folate derivative in serum is the reduced form – methyltetrahydrofolate. Serum folate levels decrease within a few days of dietary folate restriction, although tissue stores may be normal (106). Serum folate levels increase with feeding, and the use of fasting determinations has been recommended. The sensitivity of serum folate measurement for the diagnosis of clinically significant folate deficiency is uncertain; it is known that in some patients with clear-cut megaloblastic anemia caused by folate deficiency, the serum folate level is normal or only slightly low. Serum folate measurement is nonspecific; low levels are often seen in patients without other evidence of deficiency. Alcohol intake may cause a short-term decrease in serum levels in patients with adequate tissue stores. The lower limit of the reference range for serum folate varies depending on technical factors; however a serum folate concentration of less than 7 nmol/L (3 ng/mL) is commonly indicative of negative folate balance (3).

2.6 Iron supplementation during pregnancy

ID is recognized as the major cause of nutritional anemia (26). The WHO estimates that anemia resulting from ID is one of the ten most important factors contributing to the global burden of diseases (113). Pregnant women have the highest prevalence of anemia (5); therefore, it is not surprising that iron supplementation during pregnancy has been one of the most widely practiced public health measures worldwide (34).

Recently there has been debate over whether iron supplementation during pregnancy has any real impact on pregnancy and birth outcomes (34;52;114). Adding to the controversy has been concern over the possible risks of prophylactic iron supplementation among iron-replete pregnant women (115;116). The first point of contention arose in part from the results of a Cochrane systematic review that found insufficient data on the effects of iron supplementation during pregnancy, beneficial or harmful, on outcomes for the mother or her offspring (117). Similar conclusions about the lack of evidence on the impact of iron supplementation during pregnancy on maternal and infant outcomes appeared in several literature reviews (30;31;43;118). Explanations for the lack of positive findings included: examining groups with a low prevalence of anemia and a low incidence of LBW (<2500 g), inadequate sample sizes, absence of maternal and infant clinical outcomes and not identifying hematological abnormalities in the first trimester (43;114;117;118).

There have been concerns that administration of prophylactic iron supplementation may create pools of unabsorbed iron in the intestine, which could lead to a greater degree of local oxidative stress (116). The maternal Hb distribution is a U-shaped curve; infants whose mothers have a very high as well as a very low Hb concentration are at increased risk for poor health outcomes (30). Iron is a participant in the Fenton reaction, a process that results in the production of free radicals and oxidative damage (119). Over time, oxidative stress has been associated with aging, cancer and the development of cardiovascular diseases (119). While it would be difficult for reproductive aged women to become iron overloaded because of menstrual blood loss, moderately elevated iron stores have been shown to increase Type 2 diabetes (120). Concern has centered around the possibility that prophylactic iron supplementation may increase risk when the mother is not anemic or ID (27).

The advisability of routine iron supplementation during pregnancy, regardless of whether the mother is anemic, has been heavily debated in the United States (51;121). The US Preventive Services Task Force released a statement that present evidence was insufficient for it to either recommend or not recommend routine use of iron supplements in pregnant women with a Hb concentration $\geq$ 100 g/L (121). Two RCTs were conducted in the US to examine the benefits of prophylactic iron supplementation during pregnancy (122;123). The results of these trials (122;123), in addition to a large double-blinded cluster RCT conducted in Nepal (124), indicate that prophylactic iron supplementation is beneficial for improving infant outcomes, and importantly, that initiating iron supplementation early in pregnancy may be a critical requirement for its observed effectiveness (**Table 2.6**).

Across the three studies, iron supplementation was initiated between 9 and 12 weeks of gestation and no later than 20 weeks of gestation. The studies in Ohio and North Carolina randomized mothers to either 30 or 0 mg of Fe as ferrous sulfate per day (122;123). The large double-blinded RCT in Nepal examined five treatment arms; two of which included folic acid (400 μg) and the combination of iron (60 mg of ferrous fumarate) with folic acid (124). The control group in the Nepal study was vitamin A.

All three studies found significantly higher birth weights among infants whose mothers were randomized to iron supplements compared to controls (122-124). A lower incidence of LBW infants was found in the Ohio and Nepal study but not in North Carolina. A lower incidence of preterm deliveries was found in the two US studies but not in the Nepal study. The Nepal study was the only one to find a statistically significant difference in the incidence of small-for-gestational age infants. Iron supplements did not affect linear growth in the Nepal and North Carolina study (linear growth was not measured in the Ohio study). The Nepal study reported higher head and chest circumferences in treatment groups compared to the control.

Table 2.6

A description of studies that examine iron and folate supplementation initiated early or before pregnancy on hematological measures and pregnancy and infant outcomes.

Country: United States
Author, year: Cogswell et al. 2003 (122)

Objectives and Methods	Intervention	Outcomes	
Objectives: To examine the impact of first trimester Fe supplementation on 3rd trimester maternal anemia and infant outcomes. Design: Randomized controlled trial. Participants: 275 low-income pregnant women living in Cleveland, USA who were <20 wk of gestation, non-anemic (Hb ≥ 110 g/L) and iron-replete (ferritin ≥ 40 µg/L). Gestational age at baseline: 10.9 ±3.5 weeks of gestation in iron supplement group and 10.6 ±4.1 weeks of gestation in the control group.	Treatment groups: 30 mg Fe as ferrous sulfate or 0 mg Fe per day. Length of supplementation: a) Participants were assigned Fe or placebo from study entry until 28 weeks gestation. Randomization ended at 28 weeks gestation. b) From 29-38 weeks of gestation women in treatment group remained on 30 mg Fe unless iron stores were absent, in which case they were given 60 mg Fe c) From 29-38 weeks of gestation women in control group continued with placebo if they were non-anemic and replete, or were assigned 30 mg Fe if they were non-anemic and iron depleted; or were assigned 60 mg Fe if they had absent iron stores.	Maternal iron status measured at 28 weeks of gestation: a) Hb, ferritin, mean cell volume, erythrocyte protoporphyrin b) Anemia (Hb<110 g/L) Infant outcomes: a) Birth weight, birth length, gestational age b) Low birth weight (< 2500 g), preterm births (<37 wk of gestation), low birth weight infants born at term, (≥37 wk of gestation and <2500 g), small-for gestational age (defined as <10th percentile of weight at birth for gestational age)	Compa supple signifi 1) 2) 3) No sig in: 1) 2) 3)

Table 2.6 – Cont'd

Country: United States
Author, year: Siega-Riz et al. 2006 (123)

Objectives and Methods	Intervention	Outcomes	
Objectives: To examine the impact of first trimester Fe supplementation on 3rd trimester maternal anemia and infant outcomes. Design: Randomized controlled trial. Participants: 429 low-income pregnant women living in North Carolina, USA who were <20 wk of gestation, non-anemic (Hb ≥ 110 g/L) and iron-replete (ferritin ≥ 40 µg/L). Gestational age at baseline: 12.3 ±2.6 weeks of gestation in iron supplement group and 12.4 ±2.9 weeks of gestation in the control group.	Treatment groups: 30 mg Fe as ferrous sulfate or 0 mg Fe per day. Length of supplementation: a) Participants were assigned Fe or placebo from study entry until 28 weeks gestation. Randomization ended at 29 weeks gestation. b) From 29-32 weeks of gestation women received the clinic's prenatal supplement, which contained at least 30 mg of iron.	Maternal iron status measured at 26-29 weeks of gestation: a) Hb, ferritin b) Anemia (Hb<110 g/L) Infant outcomes: a) Birth weight, gestational age b) Low birth weight (< 2500 g), preterm births (<37 wk of gestation) and small-for gestational age (<10th percentile of birth weight for gestational age by sex- and race-specific standards)	Compared to supplements significantly: 1) High infan gram 2) Low (7.5% No significar 1) Mate trime 2) Prop 3rd tr 3) Mear deliv 4) Prop 5) Smal p=0.:

Table 2.6 – Cont'd

Country: Nepal
Author, year: Christian et al. 2003 (124)

Objectives and Methods	Intervention	Outcomes	
Objectives: To examine the additional impact of first trimester multiple micronutrient supplementation over Fe alone on 3rd trimester maternal anemia and infant outcomes. Design: Double blinded cluster randomized controlled trial. Participants: 4926 non-pregnant married women living in south eastern Nepal were followed from the time pregnancy was ascertained until 2-3 months postpartum. Gestational age at baseline: 11.3 ±5.1 weeks of gestation in iron supplement group and 11.2 ±5.1 weeks of gestation in the control group.	Treatment groups: 30 villages were divided into sectors. Sectors were randomly assigned to 1 of 5 treatment arms: 1. Control group was Vitamin A (1000 µg retinol equivalents as retinol acetate) 2. Vitamin A and 400 µg of folic acid; 3. Vitamin A, folic acid and 60 mg of Fe as ferrous fumarate 4. Vitamin A, folic acid, iron and 30 mg of zinc 5. Vitamin A, folic acid, iron, zinc and 11 other nutrients each at the approximate recommended daily allowance for pregnancy. 6. Length of supplementation: Participants were assigned supplement treatment groups from study entry until up to 12 weeks after a live birth and ≥ five weeks after a miscarriage or stillbirth.	Maternal iron status measured at 32 weeks of gestation: a) Hb, ferritin, iron b) Severe anemia (Hb<70 g/L), mild-to-moderate anemia (Hb 70-109 g/L, any anemia (Hb<110 g/L), and iron deficiency anemia (Hb < 100 g/L and ferritin <12 µg/L). Infant outcomes: a) Birth weight, length, chest circumference, head circumference b) Low birth weight (< 2500 g), preterm births (<37 wk of gestation) and small-for-gestational age (below 10th percentile of US national reference for fetal growth) (125).	Compared to pl in the first trime 1) Higher ferritin (p=0.0 concen 2) Lower trimest modera any an iron de p<0.00 3) Higher ± 436 v 4) Infants 2.1 cm. ±1.5 cm 5) Lower 43.4, R 6) Lower infants 0.83 to No significant c folate suppleme 1) Length 2) Propor

In the two US studies, first trimester iron supplementation improved infant outcomes even among females who were non-anemic and iron-replete at 12 weeks of gestation (122;123). In the Nepal study, a modest reduction in the incidence of LBW infants was reported among mothers supplemented with IFA vs. vitamin A. Given the poor nutritional status of Nepalese mothers at conception, it may be interpreted as remarkable that iron supplementation impacted birth weight at all.

Estimations from study control groups indicate over two fifths (43%) of babies in the Nepal study weighed less than 2500 g at birth, compared to 17% and 10% in Ohio and North Carolina, respectively. After supplementation the incidence of LBW in Nepal was 34% in the IFA group (16% reduction), 4% in Ohio (13% reduction) and 5% in North Carolina (5% reduction). The authors of the Nepal study estimated that 11 Nepalese women would need to take IFA supplements to avert one LBW baby. Globally, 15.3% of all babies are born with LBW; the prevalence is 2.5 times greater in developing (16.4%) compared to developed (6.2%) countries (11). The potential impact of IFA supplements on birth outcomes is considerable, especially in the developing world where 90% of the 250 million LBW babies are born each year (126). Across different populations, LBW infants experience 4-10 times the risk of neonatal death (127;128).

It is noteworthy to mention that the two American studies are controversial amidst recent reviews that have stated that there is insufficient evidence to support an association between iron supplementation during pregnancy and increases in birth weight (34;52;114). Both American studies reported a significantly higher mean birth weight in the group receiving iron vs. placebo;

however, neither of the studies found significant differences in third trimester Hb or ferritin concentrations or in the prevalence of anemia between mothers given placebo and those given 30 mg of iron supplementation (122;123). The results of these two US studies raise the question of how iron supplementation can increase infant birth weight without having an effect on iron status at 28 weeks of gestation.

Both of the American studies were double-blinded randomized controlled trials; however, study limitations may have influenced the final outcomes (122;123). In the Ohio study, despite randomization, women in the placebo group had significantly higher pre-pregnancy weight and initial iron stores compared to those in the treatment group (122). After adjustments for these differences, larger reductions in absent iron stores and iron deficiency anemia were found in the third trimester in the iron vs. placebo group. A large number of women were lost to follow-up in the North Carolina study (123) and the Ohio study found women who were lost to follow-up entered the study earlier in gestation and were more likely to be black compared to those who remained in the study (122).

It is possible that study limitations may not be the reason why iron supplementation did not improve iron status in the third trimester. The authors of the American studies suggest a few possible explanations for why iron supplementation significantly improved infant birth weight without effecting maternal iron status in the third trimester. One possible explanation is that iron supplements may be preferentially transferred to the fetus instead of to the mother"s iron stores (122;123). Such a mechanism for preferential transfer of iron that would influence birth weight is unknown. Other mechanisms that do not relate to iron deficiency have been postulated, such as iron supplementation improving maternal appetite, and thereby energy consumption and increased intrauterine growth or iron supplementation leading to increased plasma volume expansion. Currently, little is known about the biological mechanisms by which poor iron status may affect birth weight.

The Nepal study found a significant effect of iron supplementation on maternal iron status indicators (124). Compared to placebo, Nepalese mothers given IFA supplements from a mean of 11 weeks gestation to 32 weeks gestation had significantly higher third trimester Hb, ferritin and iron concentrations and significantly lower TfR concentrations (**Table 2.6**). Iron containing supplements reduced third trimester anemia by 36-54%. An observed effect of iron supplementation on maternal iron status indicators in the third trimester among Nepalese women may be attributable to the fact that women had very poor iron status to begin with. Iron and folic acid supplementation reduced severe anemia by 90% to a prevalence of 0.7% (124).

Few studies have examined the effect of antenatal micronutrient supplementation on changes in the biochemical status of several micronutrients during pregnancy (129). Results from the RCT in Nepal found that antenatal iron and folic acid supplementation significantly improved maternal hematologic status during pregnancy compared with placebo (130). Combinations of folic acid plus iron and zinc and folic acid plus iron, zinc and multiple micronutrients did not provide additional benefit to maternal hematological indicators compared to folic acid and iron (130). The study also found that supplementation with folic acid alone or with iron significantly decreased folate deficiency from the first to the third trimester compared to control (129). Antenatal supplementation with multiple micronutrients decreased the prevalence of serum riboflavin, vitamin B-6, vitamin B-12, folate and vitamin D deficiencies but had no effect on infection (129).

In a subsequent paper on the effects of supplementation regimens on infant mortality, the authors of the Nepal study found that IFA supplementation was associated with a 21% reduction (95% CI: - 48% to 20%) in 3 month mortality among all births and a 47% reduction in 3 month mortality (95% CI: 8%, 70%) among preterm births (131). The effect of treatment groups on birth weight was estimated in a separate paper by calculating the mean difference in birth weight between control and treatment groups (132). The shape of the birth weight distribution in the multiple micronutrient group was similar to that of the control group. Compared to the control group, the folic acid and iron group had fewer infants in the lower tail of distribution but a similar proportion in the upper tail. IFA supplementation may have improved survival due to the improvement in birth weight at the lower end of the distribution.

The results of the Nepal study provide convincing evidence that earlier initiation of iron supplementation improves maternal iron status indicators in the third trimester, increases infant birth weight, reduces preterm deliveries and reduces small-for-gestational aged infants. Results from two American studies suggest that iron supplementation started in early pregnancy may have benefits among high risk groups beyond the reduction of iron deficiency anemia during pregnancy (122;123). There are a few other studies that give support to the possibility that iron supplements are required in the first trimester to have a positive impact on infant birth outcomes. In Australia, the impact of iron supplementation (20 mg Fe/d) vs. placebo was examined among non-anemic, well-nourished women (133). The study found no significant differences in mean birth weight, percentage of LBW, or gestational age at birth (133). In contrast to the two studies in the US (122;123), iron supplementation in the Australian study was initiated at 20 weeks of gestation, at least 8 weeks later in gestation than the two US studies. In Korea, a recent study by Lee et al. compared the impact of iron supplementation initiated in the first trimester (mean of 9.1 ± 2.3 weeks of gestation) and second trimester (20 weeks of gestation) (134). Regardless of whether women received 30 or 60 mg Fe, those supplemented with iron and folic acid in the first trimester had significantly better iron status indicators in the third trimester and at delivery compared to those who started supplementation after 20 weeks gestation.

2.7 Folic acid supplementation during pregnancy

Folate plays a critical role cell division, a central feature of embryonic and fetal development (135). Folate intake is recommended throughout pregnancy to decrease the risk of poor pregnancy outcomes (48) Marginal folate nutriture during gestation can impair cellular growth and replication in the fetus or placenta (49). Low concentrations of dietary and circulating folate during pregnancy are associated with increased risk of preterm delivery, infant LBW and fetal growth retardation (48). Moreover, folate deficiency is related to elevated blood homocysteine (Hcy) concentrations, which have been associated with increased spontaneous abortion and pregnancy complications, such as placental abruption and pre-eclampsia (136).

In the periconceptional period, it is now well-recognized that folate has a protective effect against the development of neural tube defects (NTDs), specifically anencephaly and spina bifida (20;21;137). The recommended intake for females at high risk, by virtue of a previous NTD pregnancy outcome, is 4 mg/d (21). All other women capable of becoming pregnant are recommended to consume 0.4 mg of folic acid per day in addition to a folate-rich diet (138). The proportion of NTDs that can be prevented by periconceptional FA has not been established, but the general assumption is that it is probably in the area of 50–60% (137). Following the recommendations the frequency of NTDs recorded in birth defect registries of 13 (mainly Western) European countries showed no discernible improvement (139). Implementing current recommendations for preventing NTDs is challenging in developed countries, where it is estimated that 50% of pregnancies are unplanned. Malformations of NTDs occur during the fourth week of post-conception, usually before a pregnancy is confirmed (24). To be effective, all women of childbearing age need to optimize their periconceptional folate status. To address this issue, some countries have introduced mandatory folate fortification (21). Mandatory fortification has been implemented in the United States (140), Canada (111) and Chile (141). Canada began its mandatory fortification of all flour and some corn and rice products with folic acid in November 1998 (142). Cereal grain products were fortified at a level of 140 µg per 100g food in the United States and 150 µg per 100g in Canada to provide an estimated additional 100 µg of folic acid per day (49). Several studies have subsequently reported improved folate indexes (143;144) and a reduction in the frequency of NTDs by 20-30% (137;145).

2.8 The rationale for iron and folic acid vs. multiple micronutrient supplementation

Studies have shown that IFA supplementation during pregnancy significantly improves maternal hematological status and reduces the risk of poor infant outcomes (122;124;130;131;146;147) While multiple micronutrient deficiencies are common in developing countries (40;148), evidence for the benefits of multiple micronutrient (MMN) supplementation on pregnancy outcomes is sparse (30;149;150). In 1999, UNICEF/WHO/UNU recommended that MMN supplements should replace the existing IFA supplement (16). Recommendations stated that MMN supplementation should be promoted in pregnant women and adolescents in developing countries to prevent anemia and other micronutrient deficiencies and to improve stores before pregnancy (16).

Recent controlled trials among pregnant women in Mexico (147) Nepal (124) and West Africa (128) did not find any effects on birth weight of prenatal MMN supplementation in addition to the effect of IFA. A study among non-pregnant adolescent females in Bangladesh found twice weekly MMN supplements improved the status of micronutrients that were assessed but was not more efficacious that IFA supplementation alone in improving hemoglobin (Hb) and iron status (151). Supplements contained 120 mg elemental Fe as ferrous sulfate, 3.5 mg of folic acid and 2.42 mg vitamin A (retinol) as retinyl palmitate and were provided for a total duration of 12 weeks. One explanation for why MMN supplements may not be as efficacious as iron alone in reducing anemia or ID (146;147;151) is that nutrients other than iron in the MMN formulation, such as zinc and magnesium, may interfere with the absorption of iron (152).

Moreover, there is concern that MMN supplementation may increase mortality risk among term infants (131). In a large-scale double-blinded RCT in Nepal, MMN supplementation had the largest effect on birth weight (increase of 64 g; 95%CI: 12, 115) (124). MMN supplementation did not show any significant reductions in mortality; whereas, mothers who received folic acid alone or with iron showed increased survival among infants (131). Folic acid and iron was associated with an overall 21% reduction (95% CI: 48% reduction to increase of 20%), and a 47% reduction in 3 month mortality (95% CI: 8%, 70%) among preterm births. One explanation for slightly elevated risk of early infant mortality (RR: 1.07, 95% CI: 0.75, 1.58), especially among term births (RR: 1.74, 95% CI: 1.00, 3.04) in the MMN group is the disproportionately higher rate of high birth weight (≥3.3 kg) among term infants whose mother received MMN supplements compared to those in the control group (124). Specifically among term infants, MMN supplementation led to a significantly higher birth weight (RR: 1.71: 95% CI: 1.10, 2.65) compared to control (vitamin A alone) (124). Higher birth rate was associated with increased risk of birth asphyxia (RR: 1.49; 95% CI: 1.04, 2.13) (131). Risk of birth asphyxia was higher among term infants whose mothers received MMN supplementation compared to controls. While MMN supplementation improved survival among the preterm infants (RR: 0.70; 95% CI: 0.41, 1.17), it also appeared to increase high birth weight and the associated risk of birth asphyxia, a known cause of perinatal mortality among the term infants (124).

In a subsequent analysis of the birth weight distribution, authors of the Nepal study found that the shape of the birth weight distribution in the MMN group was similar to that of control group, except that the location of the distribution had shifted (132). The folic acid and iron group had fewer infants in the lower tail of the distribution; however there was a similar proportion in the upper tail of the distribution compared to the control group (132). In developing countries it may be more important to influence the lower rather than the upper part of the birth weight distribution. In fact, increasing birth weights in the upper tail of the distribution may have harmful effects. The MMN group appeared to have no effect on survival because deaths averted in the smaller infants were negated by higher mortality at the upper end of the distribution (132).

2.9 Periconceptional iron and folate (IFA) supplementation

There is a growing movement in maternal and child health advocating for a focus on the periconceptional period; the period from before conception to early pregnancy (22;45;58;69). An association between periconceptional folate supplementation and reduction in neural tube defects is already well-established (20;21). Attention is now being given to whether including iron supplementation during the periconceptional period may complement iron supplementation programs during pregnancy aimed at improving maternal and infant outcomes (22). Only a few trials have demonstrated that iron supplementation during pregnancy reduces the incidence of low birth weight infants (122-124). Unlike previous trials, all of these positive studies initiated iron supplementation much earlier in pregnancy relative to those that found no improvement. This finding suggests that there is either a critical period for intervention or a need for longer duration of treatment.

In addition to strengthening antenatal programs, there is a growing recognition that it is necessary to improve iron status before pregnancy (22;45;58;69). High rates of anemia and ID among pregnant women mean that many women in developing countries enter pregnancy with low or depleted iron stores (58). Current data suggest that in developed world settings, ~50% of women do not have adequate iron storage to meet pregnancy requirements, which means they are likely to become anemic or iron deficient to some degree (93). It has only been recently that studies have started to examine preconception anemia and iron status in young women (153-156). This small number of studies have been conducted in South Asian countries where anemia rates are high and many females conceive shortly after marriage, making it easier to identify females during the periconceptional period (154-156).

A recent study in Anhui, China examined the relationship between preconception Hb, ferritin, and B-vitamin status and pregnancy outcome in apparently healthy women (156). Previous to the study, the authors had reported a high prevalence of B-vitamin deficiencies, anemia, and depleted iron stores in a cohort of young Chinese textile workers who were planning to become pregnant (155). The prospective study was the first of its kind to report an association between preconception maternal anemia and ferritin status and adverse pregnancy outcomes (156). Preconception maternal anemia was significantly associated with infant growth, including birth weight and the risk of LBW. The mean birth-weights of infants born to women with mild and moderate anemia were 144 and 199 g lower, respectively, than those of infants born to women without preconception anemia. Women with moderate anemia before conception were 6 times as likely to deliver a LBW infant and 5 times more likely to have an infant with fetal growth restriction.

Although anemia was an important predictor of pregnancy outcome, preconception IDA was shown to have a particularly strong effect on birth-weight. Infants born to women with preconception IDA and adequate B-vitamin status weighed on average 241 g less than those born to women without anemia. It is uncertain whether infant growth deficits resulted from already anemic females developing more severe anemia during pregnancy or if anemia in the periconceptional period has an independent effect on infant growth. However, both scenarios indicate that female periconceptional anemia and iron status are important determinants of pregnancy outcomes.

In Indonesia, a program aimed at providing affordable IFA tablets to pregnant women found 45.2% of pregnant women were suffering from anemia (154). The high prevalence of anemia among pregnant women motivated the Indonesian Ministry of Health (MOH) to promote IFA supplements for female workers and school girls. The study describes preliminary results from a pilot program implemented by the MOH and MotherCare that targeted anemia control to newly-wed women. As part of an already existing program to counsel couples about marriage and require them to obtain a tetanus toxoid immunization before obtaining a marriage certificate, women were also counseled to buy and take 30-60 IFA tablets (60 mg elemental iron and 0.25 mg folic acid). Over the course of the 3-4 month program, the prevalence of anemia decreased from 23.8% to 14.0% (154).

In Bangladesh, a study was conduced among young nulliparous women to examine the effectiveness of IFA supplementation (120 mg elemental Fe as ferrous sulfate, and 3.5 mg folic acid) on hematologic indices before pregnancy (157). The study was conducted among urban adolescent (14-19 years old) garment workers. Compared to placebo, weekly IFA supplements significantly reduced the prevalence of anemia and ID by 91% and 93%, respectively. However, after 3 months of IFA supplementation a sizeable proportion of women remained deficient; 30% were anemic and 65% had depleted iron stores.

Community-based studies to compare daily vs. weekly IFA supplementation programs have recently been conducted in Cambodia, Vietnam and the Philippines among women of reproductive age (153). In Cambodia, 6 months of weekly IFA supplements improved Hb concentrations among schoolgirls but not among factory workers or women living in rural areas

(158). In the Philippines, serum ferritin concentrations were higher by 20.4 ± 2.2 µg/L in women who took IFA tablets compared to those who did not; there were no significant differences observed in Hb concentrations (159). In Vietnam, 12 months of weekly IFA supplementation decreased the prevalence of anemia from 46% to 19% and ID from 8.9% to 5.1% among non-pregnant women (160). While the efficacy of weekly IFA supplementation has yet to be determined, it poses a potential strategy for improving coverage of at-risk populations in developing countries where resources are limited.

2.10 Conclusion

Currently, there is an emerging movement towards implementing IFA supplementation to women before pregnancy (22). Conventionally, strategies to control and treat anemia during pregnancy have focused on providing IFA supplements to pregnant women through maternal and child health care programs (43). In addition to strengthening antenatal programs, there is a growing recognition for the need to improve iron status before pregnancy (69). High rates of anemia and ID among pregnant women mean that many women in developing countries enter pregnancy with low or depleted iron stores (69). Current data suggest that in developed world settings, ~50% of women do not have adequate iron storage to meet pregnancy requirements, which means they are likely to become anemic or ID to some degree (93). Improving the iron and folate status of women before pregnancy incorporates a life cycle approach to maternal and infant health.

There is a lack of data to support positive and long-term effects of periconceptional care on both the mother and the child (69). It has only been recently that studies have started to examine preconception anemia and iron status in young women (153-156). These studies have been conducted in South Asian countries where anemia rates are high and many women conceive shortly after marriage, making it easier to identify women during the periconceptional period (153-156). This handful of studies have reported promising results of the impact of periconceptional IFA supplementation on hematological status (154;158-160) before and during pregnancy; however indications of improved maternal iron status during pregnancy and improved infant growth outcomes have yet to be determined.

www.ingramcontent.com/pod-product-compliance
Lightning Source LLC
Chambersburg PA
CBHW081301180526
45170CB00007B/2515